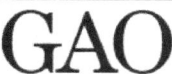

I0415893

June 2012

INDIAN HEALTH SERVICE

Action Needed to Ensure Equitable Allocation of Resources for the Contract Health Service Program

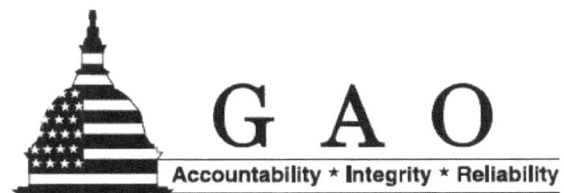

GAO

Accountability * Integrity * Reliability

GAO-12-446

GAO
Accountability * Integrity * Reliability

Highlights

Highlights of GAO-12-446, a report to congressional addressees

INDIAN HEALTH SERVICE

Action Needed to Ensure Equitable Allocation of Resources for the Contract Health Service Program

Why GAO Did This Study

IHS, an agency in the Department of Health and Human Services (HHS), provides health care to American Indians and Alaska Natives. When care at an IHS-funded facility is unavailable, IHS's CHS program pays for care from non-IHS providers if the patient meets certain requirements and funding is available. The Patient Protection and Affordable Care Act requires GAO to study the administration of the CHS program, including a focus on the allocation of funds. IHS uses three primary methods to determine the allocation of CHS funds to the 12 IHS geographic area offices: base funding, which accounts for most of the allocation; annual adjustments; and program increases, which are provided to expand the CHS program. GAO examined (1) the extent to which IHS's allocation of CHS funding varied across IHS areas, and (2) what steps IHS has taken to address funding variation within the CHS program. GAO analyzed IHS funding data, reviewed agency documents and interviewed IHS and area office officials.

What GAO Recommends

GAO suggests that Congress consider requiring IHS to develop and use a new method to allocate all CHS program funds to account for variations across areas, notwithstanding any restrictions now in federal law. GAO also recommends, among other things, IHS use actual counts of CHS users in methods for allocating CHS funds. HHS concurred with two of GAO's recommendations, but did not concur with the recommendation to use actual counts of CHS users. GAO believes that its recommendation would provide a more accurate count of CHS users.

View GAO-12-446. For more information, contact Kathleen M. King at (202) 512-7114 or kingk@gao.gov.

What GAO Found

The Indian Health Service's (IHS) allocation of contract health services (CHS) funds varied widely across the 12 IHS geographic areas. In fiscal year 2010, CHS funding ranged from nearly $17 million in one area to more than $95 million in another area. Per capita CHS funding for fiscal year 2010 also varied widely, ranging across the areas from $299 to $801 and was sometimes not related to the areas' dependence on CHS inpatient services, as determined by the availability of IHS-funded hospitals. The allocation pattern of per capita CHS funds has been generally maintained from fiscal year 2001 through fiscal year 2010. This is due to the reliance on base funding—which incorporates all CHS funding from the prior year to establish a new base each year—and accounts for the majority of funding. In fiscal year 2010, when CHS had its largest program increase and base funding was the smallest proportion of funding for any year, base funding still accounted for 82 percent of total CHS funds allocated to areas. Further, allocations of program increase funds are largely dependent on an estimate of CHS service users that is imprecise. IHS counts all users who obtained at least one service either funded by CHS or provided directly from an IHS-funded facility during the preceding 3-year period. This count therefore includes an unknown number of individuals who received IHS direct care only and who had not received contract health services.

IHS has taken few steps to evaluate funding variation within the CHS program and IHS's ability to address funding variations is limited by statute. IHS officials told GAO that the agency has not evaluated the effectiveness of base funding and the CHS Allocation Formula. Without such assessments, IHS cannot determine the extent to which the current variation in CHS funding accurately reflects variation in health care needs. While IHS has formed a workgroup to evaluate the existing formula for allocating program increases, the workgroup recommended, and the Director of IHS concurred, that the CHS Allocation Formula for distributing program increases would not be evaluated until at least 2013. The workgroup members maintained that the CHS program had only begun receiving substantial increases in fiscal years 2009 and 2010, and the full impact of these increases needed to be reviewed before making recommendations to change the formula. However, GAO found that IHS has used the formula to allocate program increases, at least in part, in 5 years since 2001. GAO also concluded that, because of the predominant influence of base funding and the relatively small contribution of program increases to overall CHS funding, it would take many years to achieve funding equity just by revising the methods for distributing CHS program increase funds. Further, federal law restricts IHS's ability to reallocate funding, specifically limiting reductions in funding for certain tribally-operated programs, including some CHS programs, and imposing a congressional reporting requirement for proposed reductions in base funding of 5 percent or more. According to IHS officials, no such IHS proposal to reallocate base funding has ever been transmitted to the Congress.

Contents

Abbreviations

CHS	Contract Health Services
HHS	Department of Health and Human Services
IHS	Indian Health Service

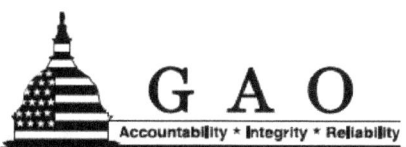

United States Government Accountability Office
Washington, DC 20548

June 15, 2012

Congressional Addressees

Adequate access to health care services for American Indians and Alaska Natives, including equitable access to care for those living in different geographic areas, has been a long-standing concern.[1] The Indian Health Service (IHS) within the Department of Health and Human Services (HHS) is the federal agency overseeing health care services to approximately 1.9 million American Indians and Alaska Natives. Direct care services are those provided directly at hospitals, health centers, or health stations that may be federally or tribally operated[2] and are located in 12 federally designated geographic areas overseen by IHS area offices.[3] When services are not accessible or available at an IHS or tribal facility, IHS or the tribes may purchase them from other providers through the Contract Health Services (CHS) program. The CHS program is administered at the local level by individual CHS programs generally affiliated with IHS-funded facilities in each area.[4] These individual CHS programs may be federally or tribally operated.

---

[1]For example, see GAO, *Indian Health Service: Health Care Services Are Not Always Available to Native Americans*, GAO-05-789 (Washington, D.C.: Aug. 31, 2005); and *Examining Tribal Programs and Initiatives Proposed in the President's Fiscal Year 2011 Budget, Before the Committee on Indian Affairs*, 111th Congress 10 (2010) (statement of Yvette Roubideaux, Director, Indian Health Service).

[2]Under the Indian Self-Determination and Education Assistance Act, as amended, federally recognized Indian tribes can enter into self-governance compacts or self-determination contracts with the Secretary of HHS to take over administration of IHS programs provided for the benefit of Indians and because of their status as Indians and previously administered by IHS on their behalf. Self-governance compacts allow tribes to consolidate and assume administration of all programs, services, activities, and competitive grants administered by IHS, or portions thereof, while self-determination contracts allow tribes to assume administration of a program, programs, or portions thereof. *See* 25 U.S.C. §§ 450f(a) (self determination contracts), 458aaa-4(b)(1) (self-governance compacts).

[3]IHS's 12 areas are Aberdeen, Alaska, Albuquerque, Bemidji, Billings, California, Nashville, Navajo, Oklahoma City, Phoenix, Portland, and Tucson.

[4]For purposes of this report, we use the term "individual CHS program" to refer to an organizational unit that IHS calls an "operating unit," "service unit," or "facility."

Funding for the CHS program increased from $498 million in fiscal year 2005 to $779 million in fiscal year 2010. CHS funds are allocated to each of the 12 area offices, which then allocate those funds to about 66 individual federally administered CHS programs and about 177 individual tribally operated CHS programs.[5] IHS allocates the majority of CHS funds to the IHS area offices as "base funding," in which the IHS area offices distribute to each individual CHS program the same amount of CHS funds as they did in the previous year.[6] Since the 1980s, we have reported that IHS's base funding method contributes to funding disparities and inequities. For example, in 1982, we recommended that IHS abandon its reliance on base funding in order to distribute its funds more equitably; IHS did not agree with the recommendation.[7] Similarly, in 1991, we suggested that the Congress should consider requiring IHS to distribute its funds with methods that give greater weight to measures of need; the Congress has not acted on our suggestion.[8]

Some IHS areas and individual CHS programs have the resources to support more health care services than others. For example, in a recent report we found that some federal CHS programs we surveyed were able to pay for all eligible CHS services in fiscal year 2009, while other programs reported that they were unable to fund even all of the highest-priority services for the full fiscal year.[9] Similarly, IHS has found substantial differences across areas with its own measure of health care

---

[5]Congress has placed restrictions on the requirements that agencies may impose on tribes carrying out self-determination contracts or self-governance compacts. (*See* 25 U.S.C. §§ 450k(a) (self-determination contracts) and 458aaa-16 (self-governance compacts).) Consequently, tribally operated CHS programs are not generally subject to the same policies, procedures, and reporting requirements as federal CHS programs.

[6]Federally operated CHS programs receive allocations of funds which authorize obligations and tribally operated CHS programs receive lump sum payments. In this report, we refer to both these allocations and these payments as distributions of funds by the area offices.

[7]GAO, *Indian Health Service Not Yet Distributing Funds Equitably Among Tribes*, GAO/HRD-82-54 (July 2, 1982).

[8]GAO, *Indian Health Service: Funding Based on Historical Patterns, Not Need*, GAO/HRD-91-5 (Feb. 21, 1991).

[9]We also found that IHS did not have accurate data on deferrals and denials for CHS services from which to estimate funding needs for the CHS program. GAO, *Indian Health Service: Increased Oversight Needed to Ensure Accuracy of Data for Estimating Contract Health Services*, GAO-11-767 (Washington, D.C.: Sept. 23, 2011).

resources, the Federal Disparity Index. The index is intended to estimate health care resources available from all sources (including other sources of health care funding such as private health insurance and Medicare or Medicaid) and account for differences in health care needs across the areas. In fiscal year 2010, the index estimated that resources available in the most well-resourced of its 12 areas, relative to their need, were nearly 50 percent higher than in the least-resourced area and that the most well-resourced individual CHS programs had resources more than three times greater than that of the programs with the least resources.

In 2001, the Director of IHS commissioned a CHS workgroup to develop a CHS formula to allocate funding increases above base funding amounts equitably across IHS areas according to variations in need (such as health care costs and access to services) across individual CHS programs. This workgroup reported a wide range in dependence on CHS for IHS-funded medical services among IHS areas. It cited examples of two areas in which CHS eligible patients were totally reliant on CHS for inpatient care,[10] and two additional areas where CHS eligible patients had very limited direct care options for inpatient services. In contrast, IHS officials reported that as few as 10 percent of potential CHS users actually used CHS services in two other areas.

The Patient Protection and Affordable Care Act required GAO to examine the administration of the CHS program, including the allocation of funds.[11] Based on discussions with the committees of jurisdiction, we agreed to focus on IHS's allocation of CHS program funds to IHS area offices. In this report, we examined (1) the extent to which IHS's allocation of CHS funding varied across IHS areas, and (2) what steps IHS has taken to address funding variation within the CHS program.

To determine the extent to which CHS funding changed over time, we obtained and analyzed CHS allocation data from IHS for fiscal years 2001 through 2010. To determine the extent to which the IHS funding allocation varied across IHS areas, we obtained and analyzed CHS and direct care

---

[10]These two areas do not have an inpatient IHS hospital.

[11]Patient Protection and Affordable Care Act, Pub. L. No. 111-148, § 10221, 124 Stat. 119, 935 (2010) (enacting S. 1790 as reported by the S. Comm. on Indian Affairs of the Senate in December 2009 into law with amendments); S. 1790, 111th Cong. §§ 137, 199 (as reported by S. Comm. on Indian Affairs. Dec. 16, 2009).

funding allocation data from IHS for fiscal years 2001 and 2010. For these years, we also obtained IHS's active user population estimates, which IHS defines as all individuals who received at least one direct care or contract care inpatient stay, outpatient, ambulatory, or dental care service during the preceding 3-year period. We used these data to calculate per capita CHS and direct care funding for each of the IHS areas. To examine IHS efforts to address funding variations within the CHS program, we reviewed IHS documents and interviewed IHS, area and tribal officials familiar with IHS efforts to address CHS funding variations. To determine the reliability of the data provided by IHS, we reviewed IHS summary CHS allocation reports for fiscal years 2001 through 2010 and data on the IHS user population used during fiscal years 2001 and 2010, and examined consistency in terms of base funding and the application of program increases. We also discussed the data with IHS officials, and discussed CHS data with officials from six IHS area offices.[12] We determined that the IHS data were sufficiently reliable for our purposes.

To address the extent to which funding varied and what steps IHS has taken to address that variation, we also reviewed IHS policies and procedures in its *Indian Health Manual* for monitoring the allocation of CHS program funds to area offices and then to individual CHS programs. The *Indian Health Manual* is the reference for IHS employees regarding IHS-specific policy and procedural instructions for the delivery of health care services to American Indians and Alaska Natives.[13] We compared these policies and procedures to the standards described in *Standards for Internal Control in the Federal Government and Internal Control Management and Evaluation Tool.*[14] We reviewed documents and interviewed IHS headquarters officials about how base funding was

---

[12]We selected a judgmental sample of six IHS areas using a combination of criteria such as high and low per capita CHS funding, active user population, total CHS funding, and proportion of individual CHS programs with access to hospitals, and geographic location. We selected the Billings, California, Nashville, Navajo, Oklahoma, and Portland area offices for interviews.

[13]Part 2, Chapter 3 of the *Indian Health Manual* contains IHS's policies and procedures for implementing the CHS program.

[14]GAO, *Standards for Internal Control in the Federal Government*, GAO/AIMD-00-21.3.1 (Washington, D.C.: Nov. 1999) and *Internal Control Management and Evaluation Tool*, GAO-01-1008G (Washington, D.C.: Aug. 2001). Internal control is synonymous with management control and comprises the plans, methods, and procedures used to meet missions, goals, and objectives.

allocated to area offices and individual CHS programs for fiscal years 2001 through 2010, how the CHS Allocation Formula was applied, and how IHS oversees the allocation of CHS funds. We also interviewed officials from six selected area offices about their methods for allocating CHS funds to individual CHS programs, oversight of allocations, and reporting of final allocations to IHS.

We conducted this performance audit from December 2010 to June 2012 in accordance with generally accepted government auditing standards. Those standards require that we plan and perform the audit to obtain sufficient, appropriate evidence to provide a reasonable basis for our findings and conclusions based on our audit objectives. We believe that the evidence obtained provides a reasonable basis for our findings and conclusions based on our audit objectives.

Background

Federal and tribal CHS programs in each of IHS's 12 areas pay for services from external providers if services are not available directly through IHS-funded facilities, if patients meet certain requirements, and if funds are available. IHS uses three primary methods—base funding, annual adjustments, and program increases—to allocate CHS funds to the area offices.

CHS Program Administration

IHS administers contract health services through 12 IHS area offices, which include all or part of 35 states where many American Indian and Alaska Natives reside. (See fig. 1.) IHS uses CHS funds to pay for services from a variety of health care providers, including hospital- and office-based providers.[15] IHS, among other things, sets program policy for and allocates CHS program funds to the area offices. The area offices distribute funds to individual federally operated and tribally operated CHS programs that purchase contract care services from outside providers.[16] There can be multiple individual CHS programs within an area. Tribes currently administer 177 of the 243 (73 percent) individual CHS programs and receive about 54 percent of IHS's funding for CHS. In addition to receiving federal funding through IHS, the tribes may provide supplemental funds to the CHS programs they administer.[17]

[15]The CHS program can purchase a wide range of health care services, including hospital care, specialty physician services, outpatient care, laboratory, dental, radiology, pharmacy, and transportation services.

[16]Area offices are also responsible for monitoring the CHS programs, establishing procedures within the policies set by IHS, and providing CHS programs with guidance and technical assistance.

[17]Unlike federal CHS programs, tribal CHS programs are able to supplement their CHS program funds with reimbursements from Medicare, Medicaid, and private insurance for services provided at tribal health care facilities. Tribal CHS programs may also supplement their CHS funding with tribal funds earned from tribal businesses or enterprises. Medicare is the federal government's health care insurance program for individuals aged 65 and older and for individuals with certain disabilities or end-stage renal disease. Medicaid is a jointly funded federal-state health care program that covers certain low-income individuals and families.

Figure 1: Counties in the 12 IHS Areas

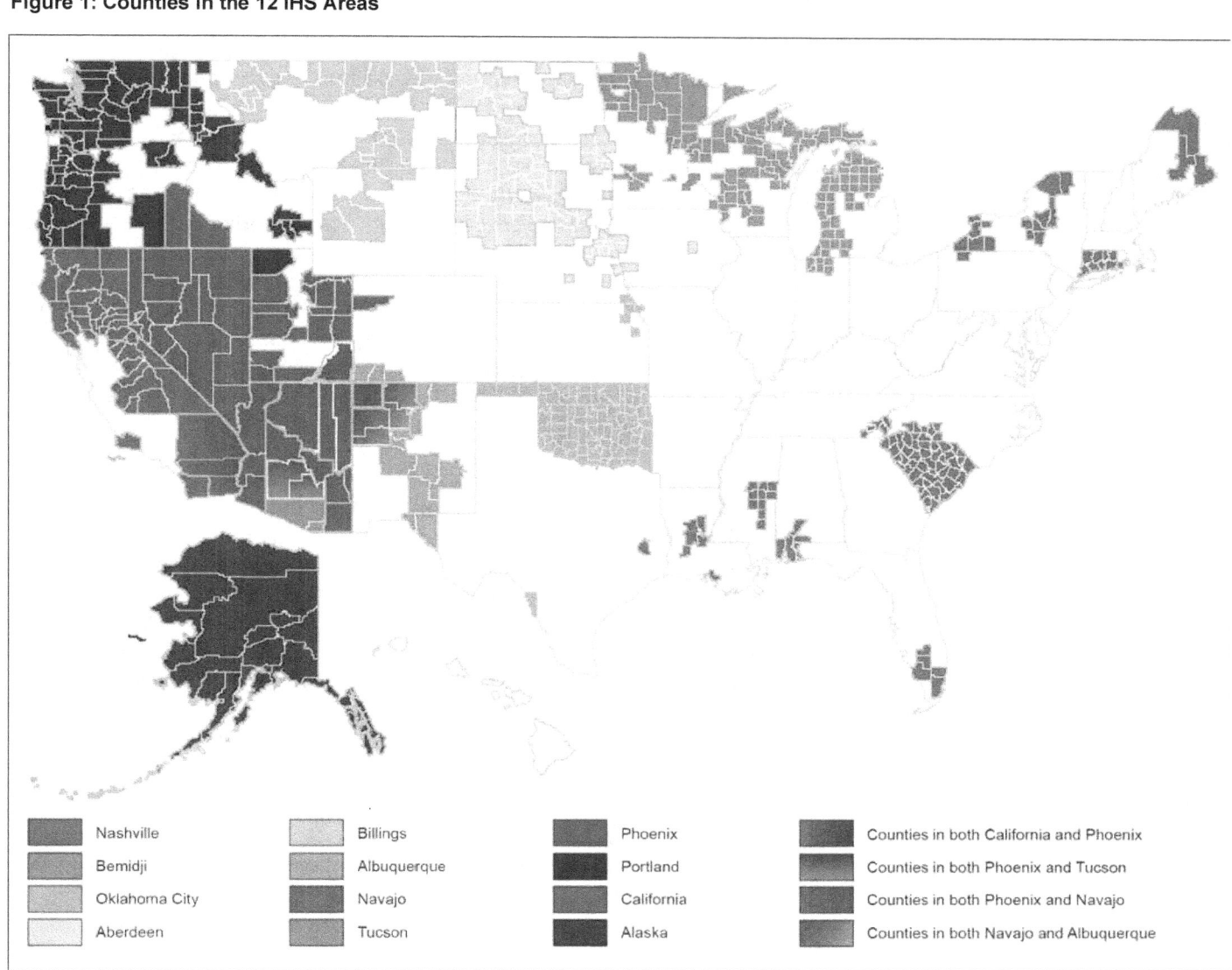

Nashville	Billings	Phoenix	Counties in both California and Phoenix
Bemidji	Albuquerque	Portland	Counties in both Phoenix and Tucson
Oklahoma City	Navajo	California	Counties in both Phoenix and Navajo
Aberdeen	Tucson	Alaska	Counties in both Navajo and Albuquerque

Source: GAO analysis of IHS information, as of July 2011.

Patients must meet certain eligibility, administrative, and medical priority requirements to have their services paid for by the CHS program. Generally, to be eligible to receive services through the CHS program, patients must reside on a reservation or within a reservation's federally established CHS Delivery Areas and be members of a tribe or tribes located on that reservation or maintain close economic and social ties with that tribe or tribes.[18] In addition, if there are alternate health care resources available to a patient, such as Medicaid and Medicare, these resources must pay for services first because the CHS program is generally the payer of last resort.[19] If a patient has met these requirements, a program committee (often including medical staff), which is part of the local CHS program, evaluates the medical necessity of the service. IHS has established four broad medical priority levels of health care services eligible for payment,[20] and each area office is required to establish priorities that are consistent with these medical priority levels. Because IHS typically does not have enough funds to pay for all CHS services requested, federal CHS programs pay first for emergency and acutely urgent medical care to the extent funds are available. They may then pay for all or only some of the lower-priority services they fund, funds permitting. Tribal CHS programs must use medical priorities when making funding decisions, but unlike federal CHS programs, they may develop a system that differs from the set of priorities established by IHS.

There are two primary paths through which patients may have their care paid for by the federal CHS program.[21] First, a patient may obtain a referral from a provider at an IHS-funded health care facility to receive services from an external provider. That referral is submitted to the CHS program for review. If the patient meets the requirements and the CHS program has funding available, the services in the referral are approved by the CHS program and a purchase order is issued to the external provider and sent to IHS's fiscal intermediary. Once the patient receives the services from the external provider, that provider obtains payment for

---

[18]See 42 C.F.R. § 136.23 (2011). The eligibility requirements for the contract care services are stricter than for direct care services. Generally, persons of Indian descent who belong to their Indian community are eligible for direct care services. See 42 C.F.R. § 136.12 (2011).

[19]See 42 C.F.R. § 136.61 (2011). There are certain exemptions to the CHS program's designation as a payer of last resort. For example, certain tribally funded insurance plans are not considered alternate resources and the CHS program must pay for care before billing the tribally funded insurance plan. See 25 U.S.C. § 1621e(f).

[20]IHS has a fifth category medical priority level for excluded services that cannot be paid for with CHS program funds, such as cosmetic plastic surgery.

[21]This describes the process by which IHS pays for services through federally operated CHS programs. Tribally operated CHS programs are not generally subject to the same policies, procedures, and reporting requirements as federal CHS programs. See 25 U.S.C. §§ 450k(a), 458aaa-16.

the services in the approved referral by sending a claim to IHS's fiscal intermediary. Second, in the case of an emergency, the patient may seek care from an external provider without first obtaining a referral. Once that care is provided, the external provider must send the patient's medical records and a claim for payment to the CHS program.[22] At that time, the CHS program will determine if the patient met the necessary program requirements and if CHS funding is available for a purchase order to be issued and sent to the fiscal intermediary. As in the earlier instance, the provider obtains payment by submitting a claim to IHS's fiscal intermediary.

In addition to funds appropriated annually for CHS, IHS also distributes funds to individual CHS programs from the Indian Health Care Improvement Fund, designed to reduce disparities and resource deficiencies at the local level as measured by IHS's Federal Disparity Index.[23] However, because these funds may be used to pay for either contract care or direct care services, it is possible that they may not finance contract care services in some programs. Further, this fund is small compared to both CHS and direct care funding. For example, in fiscal year 2010, funds distributed from the Indian Health Care Improvement Fund equaled about 6 percent of the CHS funding level, or about 2 percent of the funding level for direct care services. IHS has reported on a number of data limitations related to the current formula used to distribute funds from the Indian Health Care Improvement Fund.[24]

Methodology for Allocating CHS Funds

IHS uses three primary methods—base funding, annual adjustments, and program increases—to determine the allocation of CHS funds to the IHS area offices, which then distribute the funds to individual CHS programs.[25]

---

[22]IHS expects the external provider to seek reimbursement from any alternate resources available to the patient before submitting a claim for payment to the CHS program.

[23]See 25 U.S.C. § 1621.

[24]Indian Health Service, "A technical evaluation of the Indian Health Care Improvement Fund methodology and data" (Mar. 2010).

[25]IHS may also allocate funds from the Indian Health Care Improvement Fund that may be used for CHS services. In addition, each annual CHS appropriation identifies an amount for the Catastrophic Health Emergency Fund—a fund that IHS administers to reimburse CHS programs for their expenses from high-cost medical cases. See 25 U.S.C. § 1621a. IHS also reserves a small portion of CHS funds to pay the fiscal intermediary and for unanticipated events.

(See fig. 2.) IHS uses these methods sequentially. Base funding is the amount of CHS funds that equal the total amount of all CHS funds that each area received in the prior fiscal year. When appropriations for CHS are higher than the amount needed for base funding, IHS uses national measurements of population growth and inflation to determine annual funding adjustments. Each IHS area office receives the same percentage increase for the annual adjustments. Since 2001, when IHS has also received additional funding for what it refers to as "program increases," IHS has used the CHS Allocation Formula to determine how to allocate those program increases to the 12 area offices. According to IHS officials, IHS established the CHS Allocation Formula in part to ensure that American Indians and Alaska Natives had equitable access to contract health funds. The Allocation Formula is based on a combination of factors, including variations in the number of people using health care services, geographic differences in the costs of purchasing health care services, and access to IHS or tribally operated hospitals.

Figure 2: IHS's Primary Methods of Determining the Allocation of CHS Funds to the Area Offices

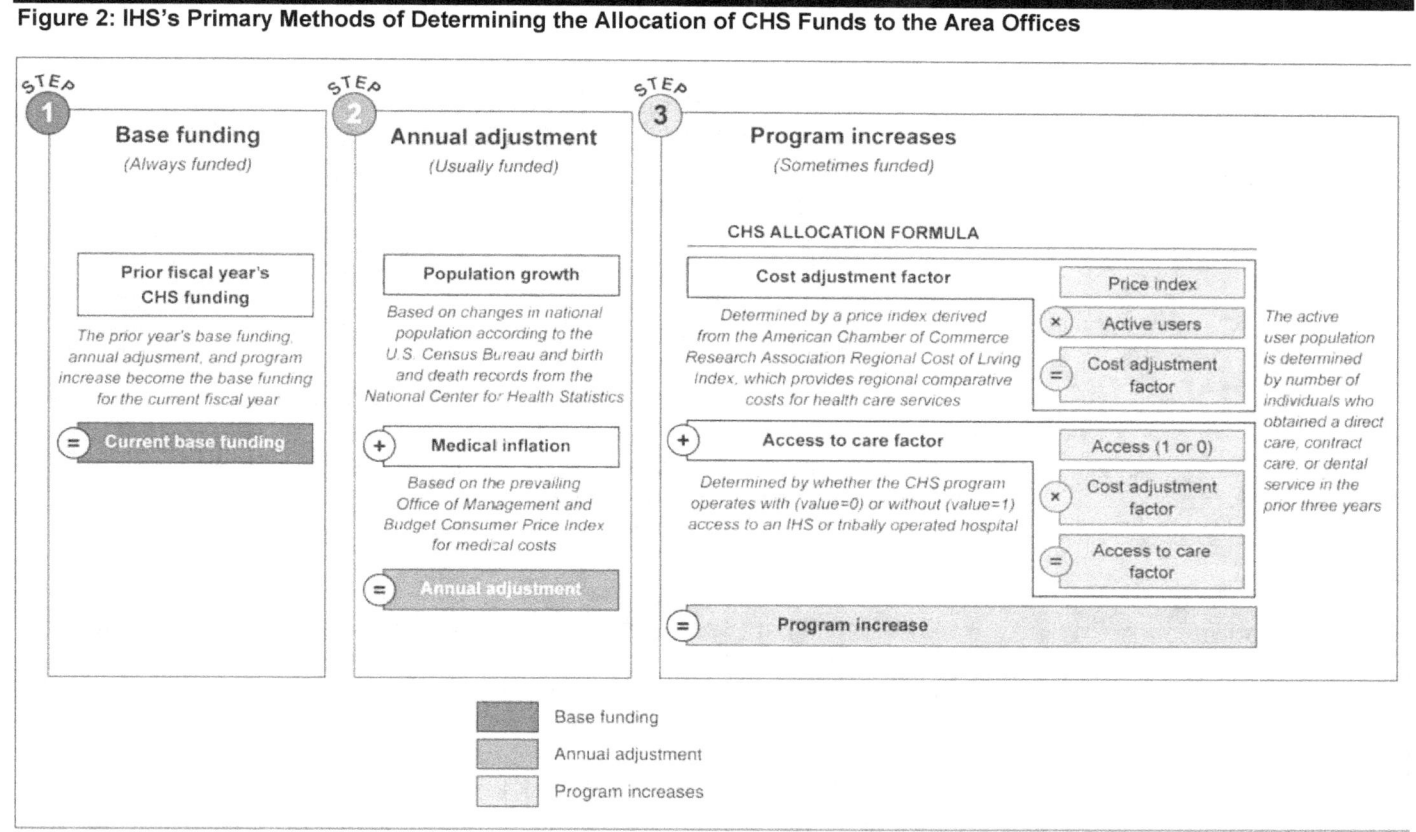

Source: GAO analysis of IHS information.

Base Funding

Most CHS funding, which IHS refers to as "base funding," is allocated based on past funding history. Each year, each of the 12 IHS area offices receives an allocation of base funding equal to the total amount of all CHS funds they received the previous fiscal year. According to IHS, base funding is intended to maintain existing levels of patient care services in all areas. Because of adjustments or funding increases that are received in most years, a new level of base funding is created in those years. IHS officials have told us they do not know the exact origins of the base funding policy, but that it dates back to the 1930s, when the health programs were under the Bureau of Indian Affairs. In 1954, Congress transferred responsibility for the maintenance and operation of hospitals and health facilities for Indians from the Bureau of Indian Affairs in the Department of the Interior to what is now IHS in HHS.[26]

Annual Adjustments

When appropriations for CHS are above the previous fiscal year's level, IHS allocates each area office an additional amount to adjust for overall population growth and inflation. The population growth funding adjustment is based on national population increases determined by the U.S. Census Bureau with annual adjustments made for changes based on state birth and death data provided by the National Center for Health Statistics. The inflation adjustment is based on the prevailing Bureau of Labor Statistics' Consumer Price Index for medical costs. IHS gives each area the same percentage increase to its base funding regardless of any population growth or cost-of-living differences among areas.[27] Typically, IHS receives increases in CHS funding that are large enough that the agency can allocate at least some for annual adjustments, even if not the full amount. The funding adjustments for population growth and inflation provided to the area offices are incorporated into the next year's base funding.

Program Increases

Additionally, in years when sufficient funding is available, IHS allocates an amount known as a program increase to each IHS area office using the CHS Allocation Formula, which it established in consultation with the tribes in 2001. IHS headquarters determines the amount allocated to an area office by applying two factors to the individual CHS programs served by that office: the cost adjustment factor, and the access to care factor. IHS determines both factors separately for each individual CHS program, and both are dependent on IHS's determination of the active user population.

- The *active user population* provides an adjustment to account for variations across individual CHS programs in the number of people using health care services. The active user population is determined by counting the number of individuals who obtained direct care services, contract care services, or dental services in the prior

---

[26]The Transfer Act of 1954, Law of Aug. 5, 1954, ch. 658 (codified at 42 U.S.C. § 2001, et seq.).

[27]In fiscal year 2009, each individual CHS program received a 1.5 percent adjustment for population growth and a 3.8 percent adjustment for inflation. In fiscal year 2010, those adjustments were 1.5 percent and 3.3 percent, respectively.

3 years. This active user population is then used as a multiplier for the cost adjustment and access to care factors.

- The *cost adjustment factor* provides an adjustment to account for geographic differences in the costs of purchasing health care services. It is based on a price index derived from the American Chamber of Commerce Researchers Association Regional Cost of Living index, which provides regional comparative costs for inpatient and outpatient services.[28] The price index for each CHS program is multiplied by the active user population for each program to determine the value of the cost adjustment factor.

- The *access to care factor* provides an additional increase only for those individual CHS programs that do not have access to an IHS or tribally operated hospital.[29] IHS area officials determine if individual CHS programs meet two qualifying criteria for this factor: (1) the individual CHS program has no IHS or tribally operated hospital with an average daily patient load of five or more, and (2) the individual CHS program does not have an established referral pattern to an IHS or tribally operated hospital within the area.[30] These additional funds are allocated to each program where there is no access to an IHS or tribally operated hospital in an amount proportional to the cost adjustment factor.

To allocate the program increase funding, IHS first designates 75 percent of the funds for increases based on the cost adjustment factor at each individual CHS program and 25 percent of the funds for the increases based on the access to care factor at each individual CHS program. IHS then totals the program increases for the individual CHS programs and allocates that total amount to the IHS area offices. Program increases allocated using the CHS Allocation Formula become part of the area offices' base funding for the next fiscal year.

---

[28]According to IHS officials, the American Chamber of Commerce Researchers Association index is used in the formula because it is maintained independently and includes data for between 270 and 350 geographical areas.

[29]Some areas have no or limited access to IHS or tribally operated hospitals so they need to purchase more services through the CHS program.

[30]IHS officials reported that an established referral pattern means that more than 50 percent of inpatient admissions go to an IHS or tribally operated hospital.

GAO-12-446 Contract Health Service Funding

IHS used the CHS Allocation Formula to allocate program increases in fiscal years 2001, 2002, and 2008 through 2010.[31] In each of those years, IHS informed the IHS area offices of the total amounts of program increase funds to be allocated to the offices and the dollar values that IHS calculated under that formula for each individual CHS program in their areas. To specifically address health care needs in local communities, IHS permits area offices, in consultation with the tribes, to distribute program increase funds to local CHS programs using criteria other than the CHS Allocation Formula. Because these adjustments are made at the individual CHS program level, they do not affect future base funding which is determined at the area level.

Allocation of CHS Funds

Funds allocated to the IHS area offices through base funding, annual adjustments, and program increases have increased substantially over the past 10 years. In fiscal year 2001, area offices received just over $386 million; in fiscal year 2010, they received just over $715 million in CHS funds.[32] (See fig. 3.)

---

[31]In fiscal years 2001 and 2002, IHS used the CHS Allocation Formula to distribute only part of the funds it received for program increases since the formula was new.

[32]Allocations to area offices are the amounts of IHS's annual CHS appropriations distributed to 12 IHS area offices at the beginning of each fiscal year. Funds allocated to area offices each year total slightly less than the amount appropriated because a portion of each annual CHS appropriation is identified for the Catastrophic Health Emergency Fund or reserved by IHS to pay for the fiscal intermediary and for unanticipated events.

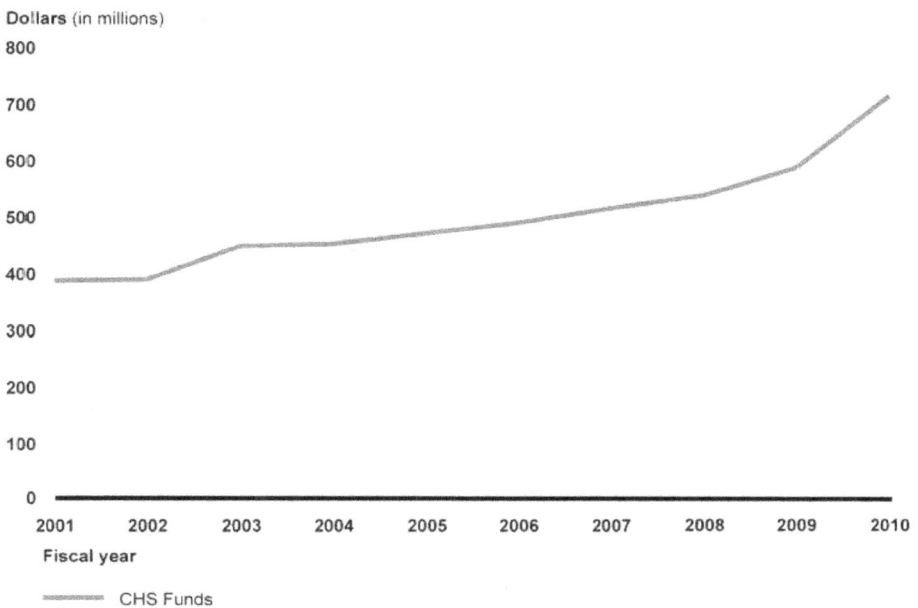

Figure 3: Total CHS Funds Allocated to IHS Area Offices, Fiscal Years 2001 through 2010

Dollars (in millions)

Source: GAO analysis of Indian Health Service data.

Note: Allocations to area offices are the amounts of IHS's annual appropriations allocated to 12 IHS area offices. Because a portion of each annual CHS appropriation is identified for the Catastrophic Health Emergency Fund or reserved by IHS to pay the fiscal intermediary and for unanticipated events, funds allocated to area offices each year total slightly less than the amount appropriated.

IHS's Allocation of CHS Funds Has Varied across IHS Areas

IHS's allocation of CHS funds has varied widely across IHS area offices, and IHS's method of allocating CHS funds has maintained those funding differences. Moreover, the CHS Allocation Formula for determining program increases uses imprecise counts of CHS users.

IHS's Allocation of CHS Funds Varied Widely across IHS Areas in Fiscal Year 2010

CHS funding varied widely across IHS area offices in fiscal year 2010. Total CHS funding for fiscal year 2010 ranged across the 12 area offices from nearly $17 million to more than $95 million. There were also substantial ranges in base funding, annual adjustments, and the program increase. For fiscal year 2010, base funding ranged from nearly $15 million to nearly $76 million, annual adjustments ranged from less than $1 million to more than $3 million, and the program increases ranged from around $1.5 million to more than $16 million across the area offices. (See table 1.)

Table 1: CHS Funding Allocated to IHS Area Offices, Fiscal Year 2010

| Area | Funds allocated to area offices, in dollars, for fiscal year 2010 | | | | IHS active user count[b] | Per capita total CHS funding, in dollars[c] |
	Base funding	Total adjustments[a]	Program increase	Total CHS funding		
Oklahoma	$75,827,291	$3,323,888	$16,114,000	$95,265,179	318,923	$299
Navajo	69,437,474	3,090,855	12,458,000	84,986,329	242,331	351
Phoenix	51,570,656	2,278,464	9,200,000	63,049,120	159,166	396
Albuquerque	29,830,959	1,327,724	6,023,000	37,181,683	85,946	433
Bemidji	41,868,282	1,865,264	8,631,000	52,364,546	102,782	509
California	31,420,785	1,400,292	7,952,000	40,773,077	78,682	518
Alaska	63,065,563	2,808,647	9,907,000	75,781,210	138,298	548
Nashville	24,243,805	2,012,527	3,899,000	30,155,332	51,491	586
Aberdeen	67,932,811	3,026,350	7,949,000	78,908,161	121,903	647
Tucson	14,805,851	658,487	1,522,000	16,986,338	25,562	665
Portland	69,230,127	3,001,723	10,985,000	83,216,850	104,097	799
Billings	49,214,400	2,193,163	5,360,000	56,767,563	70,863	801

Source: GAO analysis of IHS allocation data.

[a]Total adjustments include the inflation and population growth annual adjustments plus other adjustments IHS made.

[b]IHS uses the IHS active user count to determine the allocation of program increases. The IHS active user count includes all individuals who received at least one direct care or contract care inpatient stay or outpatient, ambulatory, or dental care service during the preceding 3-year period. For fiscal year 2010, IHS used its count of active users from fiscal year 2009 because that was the most recent year for which data were available.

[c]Per capita funding is based on the IHS active user count.

Because total funding may reflect variations in the size of the population of IHS areas, we also examined per capita funding for fiscal year 2010 using IHS's count of active users from the most recent year for which data were available.[33] Per capita CHS funding for fiscal year 2010 varied

---

[33]Per capita funding is based on IHS's count of active users in fiscal year 2009 (the most recent year for which data were available), which includes all individuals who received at least one direct care, contract care, or dental care service during the preceding 3-year period.

widely, ranging across the area offices from $299 to $801. In addition, per capita CHS funding was sometimes not related to areas' dependence on CHS for the provision of IHS-funded inpatient services. For example, California received a level of per capita funding that was in the lower half of the range for all areas, while American Indians and Alaska Natives in that area rely entirely on CHS for their IHS-funded inpatient services because there are no IHS or tribally operated hospitals. Similarly, the Bemidji area depends almost entirely on CHS for its IHS-funded inpatient services, yet received levels of per capita CHS funding that were in the lower half of the range of CHS funding for all areas.

Because CHS funds are used to purchase services not accessible or available through the direct care program, we compared patterns of funding for the direct care program and the CHS program across areas. On average, areas were allocated about three times as much in per capita direct care funding as they were in per capita CHS funding. We also found that, in general, the areas that were allocated higher amounts of per capita direct care funding were also allocated higher amounts of per capita CHS funding, and those areas that were allocated lower amounts of per capita direct care funding were also allocated lower amounts of per capita CHS funding. The notable exceptions were Alaska, which was allocated much more in per capita direct care funding than average, and Portland and Tucson, which were allocated much less in per capita direct care funding than average. Alaska was allocated per capita direct care funding ($3,340) that was about six times more than its per capita CHS funding ($548) and was the highest per capita direct care funding of all the areas, nearly double that of the area with the second highest per capita funding (Nashville, $1,869). Direct care funding for Alaska reflects the unique health care challenges that Alaska faces due to its remoteness and vast distances, which result in some of the highest costs for health care services in the United States. In contrast, the lower per capita direct care allocations to Tucson and Portland were somewhat offset by relatively higher levels of per capita CHS funding. Tucson was allocated the lowest per capita direct care funding ($1,324) but it received the third highest per capita CHS funding ($664). Similarly, Portland's per capita direct care funding ($1566) was relatively low, but its per capita CHS funding ($799), was the second highest.

In addition to variation in funding across IHS area offices, variation in funding may exist among individual CHS programs within area offices of which IHS headquarters is not aware. Some IHS area offices use methods other than the CHS Allocation Formula to distribute CHS program increases and IHS does not require the area offices to report these variations to headquarters. As a result, IHS may not be able to appropriately oversee agency operations. According to *Standards for Internal Controls in the Federal Government*, agency managers should establish appropriate and clear policies and procedures for internal reporting relationships that effectively provide managers with the information they need to carry out their job responsibilities. The standards further state that an agency must have reliable and timely communications relating to internal events to run and control its operations. IHS allows area offices, in consultation with the tribes, to distribute program increase funds to local CHS programs using different criteria than the CHS Allocation Formula to meet health care needs in local communities, but does not require that the areas inform IHS headquarters. By not requiring area offices to report to IHS headquarters about deviations in funding, IHS is not meeting internal control standards. For example, IHS headquarters officials identified two area offices that have used alternate methods to distribute CHS program increases to local CHS programs. We identified a third area that used alternative methods that IHS was not aware of, specifically using the count of actual CHS users at each individual CHS program.

IHS's Methods of Allocating CHS Funds Have Maintained Funding Differences

The allocation pattern of per capita CHS funds has been generally maintained over the 10-year period that we examined. Those areas that had the highest and the lowest levels of per capita CHS funding in fiscal year 2001 generally also had the highest and lowest levels of per capita CHS funding in fiscal year 2010. (See fig. 4.)

Figure 4: Per Capita CHS Funding in Constant Dollars, Fiscal Years 2001 and 2010, by Area

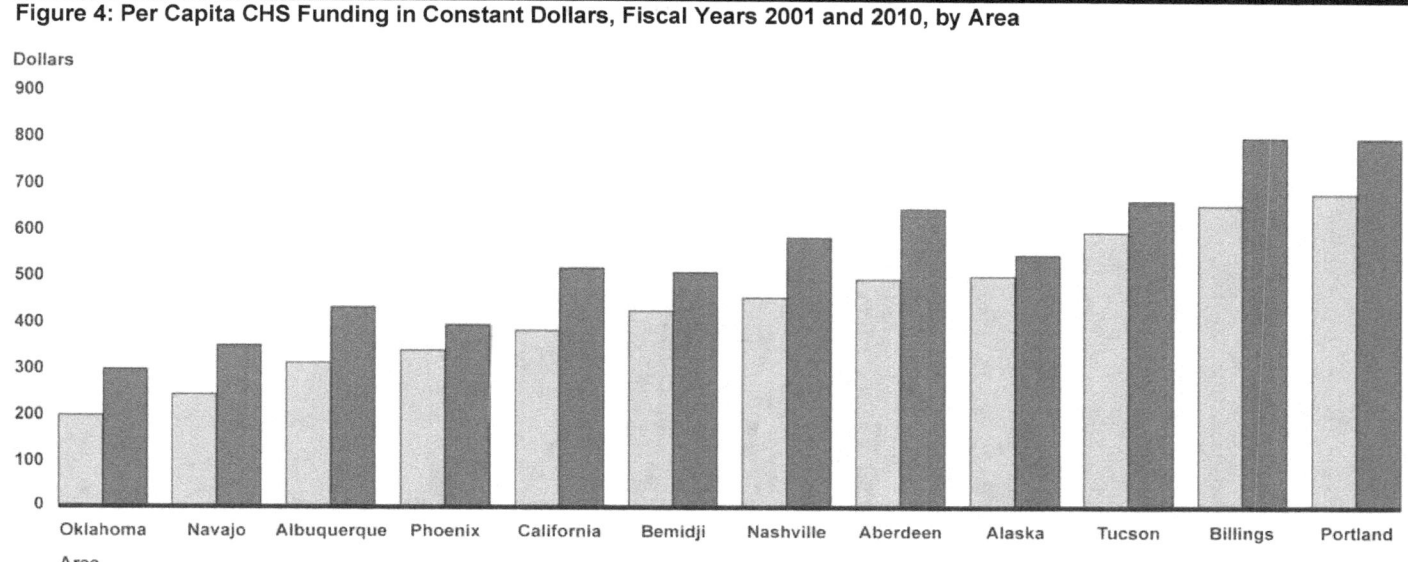

Per capita CHS funding fiscal year 2001, adjusted for inflation

Per capita CHS funding, fiscal year 2010

Source: GAO analysis of Indian Health Service data.

Note: Per capita funding is based on IHS's count of active users which includes all individuals who received at least one direct care, contract care, or dental care service during the preceding 3-year period.

Base funding, which is based solely on funding from the prior year, accounts for the great majority of CHS funds and therefore maintains any funding variations. For example, in fiscal year 2010, the year in which IHS received its largest program increase, base funding accounted for 82 percent of total CHS funds allocated to IHS area offices. (See fig. 5 for the allocation of funds in fiscal year 2010.) Annual adjustments for population growth and inflation are made as a percentage of base funding that is the same for all areas and therefore do not affect funding variations. Further, program increase funds allocated through the CHS Allocation Formula are not large enough to alter funding variations because they have been a relatively small proportion of the CHS funds that area offices receive. For example, in fiscal year 2010, CHS Allocation Formula funds amounted to about 14 percent of total CHS funding. Therefore, any variations in the original base funding amounts allocated to the areas are perpetuated since the occasional program increases are not sufficiently large to be able to close that gap.

GAO-12-446 Contract Health Service Funding

Figure 5: Allocation of CHS Funds, Fiscal Year 2010

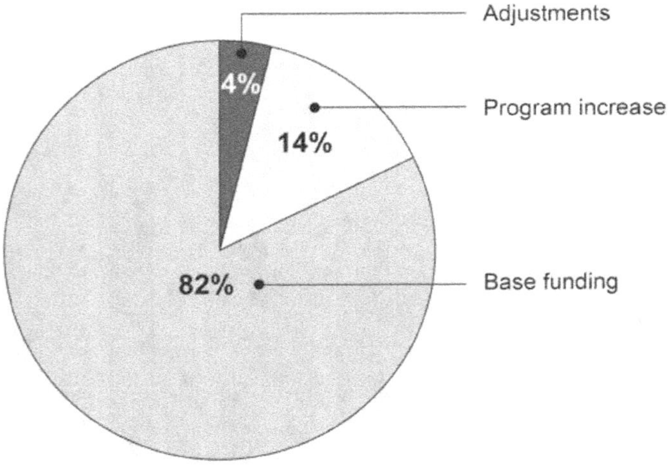

- Adjustments — 4%
- Program increase — 14%
- Base funding — 82%

Source: GAO analysis of Indian Health Service data.

The CHS Allocation Formula Uses Imprecise Counts of CHS Users to Allocate CHS Program Increases

The CHS Allocation Formula IHS uses to allocate CHS program increases to IHS area offices is largely dependent on an estimate of active users that is imprecise, even though IHS considers population estimates to be a critical factor in allocating CHS funds. In 2010, IHS's Data/Technical Workgroup noted that the active user population is not a precise measure of American Indians and Alaska Natives eligible for CHS services.[34] The CHS Allocation Formula allocates funds based on counts of all users who had at least one direct care or contract care inpatient stay, or obtained at least one outpatient, ambulatory, or dental service during the preceding 3-year period. The active user estimates that IHS used to allocate program increases therefore included an unknown proportion of patients who had not received contract health services, but rather had received only direct care services. IHS has acknowledged that its method of counting active users for the CHS Allocation Formula does not measure the number of people who actually received CHS services, nor does it measure the number of people who are eligible for CHS services. Because the active user population is used to determine

---

[34]The Data/Technical Work Group was formed to evaluate allocation of The Indian Health Care Improvement Fund and reported its findings in March 2010.

program increases, any inaccuracies in that number potentially could contribute to variation not linked to actual use of CHS services.

While IHS has an information technology system that could produce actual counts of CHS users, IHS officials do not believe that the data in the system are complete or that areas collect these data in the same way. This system contains separate tabulations of users of direct care services, contract care services, and dental care services. However, IHS officials told us that they do not provide guidance to area offices on how to record data on active CHS user counts. Nevertheless, officials from one area told us that one of their statisticians separated out the CHS users from the active user population count identified by IHS for 2 recent years and found that the CHS user count is about half of the active user population count. Without accurate data, it is not possible for IHS to know if the proportion of actual CHS users is consistent across areas.

IHS Has Taken Few Steps to Address the Funding Variation within the CHS Program

IHS has taken few steps to evaluate the funding variations within the CHS program. In addition, IHS's ability to address funding variations is limited by statute.

IHS Has Taken Few Steps to Evaluate the Funding Variations within the CHS Program

IHS has taken few steps to evaluate the funding variations within the CHS program. IHS officials told us that they have not evaluated the effectiveness of base funding and the CHS Allocation Formula in meeting the health care needs of American Indians and Alaska Natives across the IHS areas and they do not plan to do so with respect to the determination of base funding amounts. Without such assessments, IHS cannot determine the extent to which the current variation in CHS funding reflects variation in health care needs. According to *Standards for Internal Controls in the Federal Government*, agency managers should compare actual performance to planned or expected results throughout the organization and analyze significant differences. Further, the standards specify that activities need to be established to monitor performance measures and indicators.[35] IHS has not developed policies and

---

[35]GAO/AIMD-00-21.3.1.

procedures in the *Indian Health Manual* for its headquarters and field staff employees on how to conduct assessments of the CHS program funding methodologies, nor has it included goals, measures, and time frames for assessing the CHS program funding allocation performance within areas, which would potentially help IHS and the area offices identify and allocate CHS program funds to areas and local CHS programs with the greatest need.

In March 2010, the Director of IHS formed the Director's Workgroup on Improving CHS to review tribal input to improve the CHS program, to evaluate the existing formula for allocating program increases using the CHS Allocation Formula, and to recommend improvements in the way CHS business operations are conducted. The workgroup members agreed that their recommendations would apply only to program increases and not to base funding. In February 2011, the Director of IHS reported that she concurred with the four recommendations made by the workgroup in October 2010.

- The workgroup recommended that a technical subcommittee be created and charged with calculating the current CHS need and estimates of future CHS need. Such information would be essential to understanding the variation in CHS funding. However, we previously reported that IHS data on denials and deferrals that IHS used to estimate program need are incomplete and inconsistent.[36]

- The workgroup recommended convening 12 Area Work Sessions to review and make recommendations about current CHS policies and procedures, which would then be used to revise the CHS chapter of the *Indian Health Manual*, specifically relating to issues of evaluating the cost of care and communication of CHS program requirements, among others. These sessions have been completed and the workgroup is developing a summary report.

- The workgroup recommended that an evaluation of the current CHS Allocation Formula be postponed until at least fiscal year 2013. The workgroup members said that the CHS program had only begun receiving substantial increases in fiscal years 2009 and 2010, and the full impact of these increases needed to be reviewed before making recommendations to change the formula. In contrast, we found that

---

[36]GAO-11-767.

IHS has used the formula to allocate program increases, at least in part, in 5 years since 2001. Members of the workgroup we interviewed told us that outcome measures for the evaluation have not yet been defined. As part of this recommendation, they also suggested that a subcommittee be created to review the CHS Allocation Formula for equity across areas. An IHS representative to the workgroup told us that the recommendations of the subcommittee will not be considered by the full committee until the review of equity is complete.

- The workgroup recommended that the inpatient and outpatient components of the Consumer Price Index be used for any new CHS program increases that IHS may receive for fiscal year 2013 and beyond.

Members of the 2010 Director's Workgroup we spoke with expressed concern that the CHS Allocation Formula does not differentiate between large and small hospitals when determining the access to care factor, although the workgroup did not make a recommendation concerning this issue. Specifically, programs with access to small hospitals with minimal services do not receive an adjustment for access to care, and are therefore treated similarly to programs with access to large medical centers where a range of specialty care services may be available. As a result, the CHS Allocation Formula does not equitably compensate for limitations in hospital access. When the CHS Allocation Formula was created in 2001, its developers noted that the access to care factor should be refined to better reflect the complexities of the IHS system of health care. IHS has neither refined nor made any change to the way that access to care is defined.

IHS's Ability to Address Funding Variations Is Limited by Statute

Federal law restricts IHS's ability to reallocate funding should the agency desire to do so. Specifically, IHS officials identified two statutory provisions that limit IHS's ability to adjust funding allocations. The Indian Self-Determination and Education Assistance Act currently prohibits reductions in funding for certain tribally operated programs, including some CHS programs, except for limited circumstances.[37] In addition, the Indian Health Care Improvement Act imposes a congressional reporting requirement for proposed reductions in base funding for any recurring program, project, or activity of a service unit of 5 percent or more.[38] IHS officials told us that no such proposal to reallocate base funding has been transmitted to the Congress.

IHS officials have told us that areas and tribes have resisted changes to the current funding allocation methods, particularly base funding, as consistent funding allows the areas and tribes to plan and manage their resources. However, minutes from a 2010 session of the Director's workgroup show that not all tribes agree with the CHS Allocation Formula and that some workgroup members said that the current CHS Allocation Formula was not sufficiently equitable. Concerns about IHS's funding methods are longstanding. For example, in 1982, we concluded that IHS's practice of funding programs based on the previous year's funding level caused funding inequities and that IHS did not distribute funds to the neediest programs in fiscal year 1981.[39]

Conclusions

There are wide variations in CHS funding across the 12 IHS areas, and these variations are largely maintained by IHS's long-standing use of the base funding methodology. IHS officials are unable to link variations in funding levels to any assessment of health care need. As we have reported in the past and found once again in this evaluation, IHS's continued use of the base funding methodology undermines the equitable allocation of IHS funding to meet the health care needs of American Indians and Alaska Natives. Program increases for the CHS program over the years have not significantly altered variations across the areas, primarily because they are too small to have a strong impact on overall funding. Funds from the Indian Health Care Improvement Fund, designed

---

[37]The Indian Self-Determination and Education Assistance Act expressly prohibits reductions in funding in subsequent years once a required funding amount for a contract or compact is established, except for specified circumstances relating to a reduction in appropriations, congressional directive, tribal authorization, change in the amount of pass-through funds, or the completion of the activity for which funds were provided. 25 U.S.C. § 450j-1(b)(2) (relating to self-determination contracts). 25 U.S.C. § 458aaa-7(d)(1)(C)(ii) (relating to self-governance compacts).

[38]25 U.S.C. § 1680g.

[39]GAO/HRD-82-54.

to reduce funding disparities, also have had little impact because they are relatively small and not targeted solely for the CHS program. Further, federal law restricts IHS's ability to reallocate funding, principally by prohibiting reductions for certain tribally operated CHS programs, which account for more than half of total CHS funding. IHS also may be unaware of additional variation in funding across individual CHS programs because it does not require that area offices notify IHS headquarters when they choose different funding methodologies than those suggested by headquarters.

IHS can improve the equity of how it allocates program increase funds to areas through improvements in its implementation of the CHS Allocation Formula, primarily by using counts of actual CHS users rather than by using the current method of estimating the number of overall IHS users, which now includes patients who never used a CHS service, and by refining the access to care factor to account for differences in available health care services at IHS and tribally operated facilities. However, because of the predominant influence of base funding and the relatively small contribution of program increases to overall CHS funding, it would take many years to achieve funding equity just by revising the methods for distributing CHS program increase funds.

Matter for Congressional Consideration

In order to ensure an equitable allocation of CHS program funds, the Congress should consider requiring IHS to develop and use a new method to allocate all CHS program funds to account for variations across areas that would replace the existing base funding, annual adjustment, and program increase methodologies, notwithstanding any restrictions currently in federal law.

Recommendations for Executive Action

To make IHS's allocation of CHS program funds more equitable, we recommend that the Secretary of Health and Human Services direct the Director of the Indian Health Service to take the following three actions for any future allocation of CHS funds:

- require IHS to use actual counts of CHS users, rather than all IHS users, in any formula for allocating CHS funds that relies on the number of active users;

- require IHS to use variations in levels of available hospital services, rather than just the existence of a qualifying hospital, in any formula for allocating CHS funds that contains a hospital access component; and

- develop written policies and procedures to require area offices to notify IHS when changes are made to the allocations of funds to CHS programs.

Agency Comments and Our Evaluation

HHS reviewed a draft of this report and provided written comments, which are reprinted in appendix I. In its comments, HHS concurred with two of our recommendations and did not concur with one recommendation. HHS did not comment on our general findings or our conclusion that IHS's use of the base funding methodology has led to long-standing inequities in the distribution of CHS funds.

HHS concurred with our recommendation that IHS use variations in levels of available hospital services to allocate CHS funds. HHS noted that the IHS Director's Workgroup on Improving CHS will review the formula and make recommendations in fiscal year 2013. HHS also concurred with our recommendation to develop written policies to require area offices to notify IHS when changes are made in the allocations of funds to CHS programs. HHS noted that guidance requiring areas to report these changes to IHS headquarters will be added to the CHS manual; however, the agency did not specify a date for doing so.

HHS did not concur with our recommendation that it should require IHS to use actual counts of CHS users, rather than all IHS users, in any formula for allocating CHS funds that relies on the number of active users. HHS stated that IHS's combined count of all users of IHS direct care services and CHS users is intended to reflect the health care needs of those eligible for CHS services. However, as we reported, IHS's own Data/Technical Workgroup found that the current IHS active user count does not measure the number of people who are eligible for CHS services, in part because not all users of IHS direct care services are eligible for CHS services. Further, as HHS acknowledged in its comments, the current count of active users also does not reflect those who actually received CHS services. Because CHS program increases are intended to reflect variations in the numbers of CHS users among areas, we continue to believe that IHS should use counts of actual CHS users in determining program increases.

GAO-12-446 Contract Health Service Funding

We are sending copies of this report to the Secretary of Health and Human Services, Director of the Indian Health Service, appropriate congressional committees, and other interested parties. In addition, the report is available at no charge on the GAO website at http//www.gao.gov.

If you or your staffs have any questions about this report, please contact me at (202) 512-7114 or kingk@gao.gov. Contact points for our Offices of Congressional Relations and Public Affairs may be found on the last page of the report. GAO staff who made major contributions to this report are listed in appendix II.

Kathleen M. King
Director, Health Care

List of Addressees

The Honorable Daniel K. Akaka
Chairman
The Honorable John Barrasso
Ranking Member
Committee on Indian Affairs
United States Senate

The Honorable Don Young
Chairman
The Honorable Dan Boren
Ranking Member
Subcommittee on Indian and Alaska Native Affairs
Committee on Natural Resources
House of Representatives

The Honorable Jeff Bingaman
The Honorable Tim Johnson
The Honorable Lisa Murkowski
The Honorable John Thune
United States Senate

Appendix I: Comments from the Department of Health and Human Services

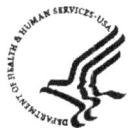

DEPARTMENT OF HEALTH & HUMAN SERVICES

OFFICE OF THE SECRETARY

Assistant Secretary for Legislation
Washington, DC 20201

MAY 22 2012

Kathleen King
Director, Health Care
U.S. Government Accountability Office
441 G Street NW
Washington, DC 20548

Dear Ms. King:

Attached are comments on the U.S. Government Accountability Office's (GAO) report entitled:
"INDIAN HEALTH SERVICE: Action Needed to Ensure Equitable Allocation of Resources for
the Contract Health Service Program" (GAO-12-446).

The Department appreciates the opportunity to review this draft section of the report prior to
publication.

Sincerely,

Jim R. Esquca
Assistant Secretary for Legislation

Attachment

**GENERAL COMMENTS OF THE DEPARTMENT OF HEALTH AND HUMAN
SERVICES (HHS) ON THE GOVERNMENT ACCOUNTABILITY OFFICE'S (GAO)
DRAFT REPORT ENTITLED, "INDIAN HEALTH SERVICE: ACTION NEEDED TO
ENSURE EQUITABLE ALLOCATION OF RESOURCES FOR THE CONTRACT
HEALTH SERVICE PROGRAM" (GAO-12-446)**

The Department appreciates the opportunity to comment on this draft report.

HHS is committed to improving the Indian Health Service's (IHS) Contract Health Services
(CHS) program and has developed the following responses to GAO's three recommendations for
executive action:

Recommendation 1:

Require IHS to use actual counts of CHS users, rather than all IHS users, in any formula for
allocating CHS funds that relies on the number of active users.

HHS Response:

We do not concur. HHS disagrees that only "actual counts of CHS users, rather than all IHS
users" should be used in the formula for the allocation of CHS funds.

1) The CHS formula is intended to reflect health care needs of American Indian and Alaska
   Native (AI/AN) populations that are eligible for CHS funds, not exclusively the sub-set
   of CHS eligible persons for which referrals were actually approved and paid during a
   given period of time. Although not all of the eligible population users will access CHS
   funds every year, almost all users will, at some time, have the need for CHS. We believe
   the active user count reflects an accurate number of defined AI/ANs who use IHS
   services over a specific period of time.

2) CHS eligible AI/ANs are a sub-set of all AI/ANs served by the IHS. The Contract Health
   Service Delivery Area residency and Tribal affiliation restrictions were adopted with
   Tribal input decades ago as a means to address inadequate CHS funding. Many Tribes
   favor less restrictive rules for measuring CHS needs and calculations used in the
   allocation formula. This view is consistent with the broad authority of the Snyder Act,
   which does not impose residency or Tribal affiliation limits. Counts of AI/AN users
   unrestricted by residency and Tribal affiliation were adopted in 2001 for the CHS
   formula following Tribal consultation. Tribal views were mixed at that time and this
   issue is expected to be reconsidered during further evaluation and Tribal consultation
   planned for 2013.

1

**GENERAL COMMENTS OF THE DEPARTMENT OF HEALTH AND HUMAN
SERVICES (HHS) ON THE GOVERNMENT ACCOUNTABILITY OFFICE'S (GAO)
DRAFT REPORT ENTITLED, "INDIAN HEALTH SERVICE: ACTION NEEDED TO
ENSURE EQUITABLE ALLOCATION OF RESOURCES FOR THE CONTRACT
HEALTH SERVICE PROGRAM" (GAO-12-446)**

Recommendation 2:

Require IHS to use variations in levels of available hospital services, rather than just the
existence of a qualifying hospital, in any formula for allocating CHS funds that contains a
hospital access component.

HHS Response:

We concur. HHS agrees the hospital access component of the allocation formula should include
variations in levels of available hospital services. The Director's Workgroup on Improving CHS
will review and discuss the complete formula and make recommendations in FY 2013.

Recommendation 3:

Develop written policies and procedures to require area offices to notify IHS when changes are
made to the allocations of funds to CHS programs.

HHS Response:

We concur. HHS agrees and policy guidance will be developed and included in the CHS manual
requiring Areas to report these changes to IHS Headquarters.

2

Appendix II: GAO Contact and Staff Acknowledgments

GAO Contact	Kathleen M. King, Director, (202) 512-7114 or kingk@gao.gov
Staff Acknowledgments	In addition to the contact named above, Martin T. Gahart (Assistant Director), George Bogart, Carolyn Feis Korman, and Laurie Pachter made key contributions to this report.

www.ingramcontent.com/pod-product-compliance
Lightning Source LLC
Chambersburg PA
CBHW080933290526
45795CB00007BA/2738